MANUAL OF PROSTATE CANCER

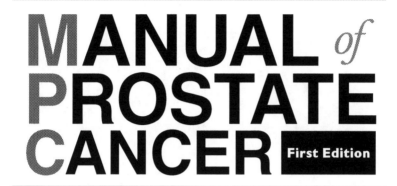

MANUAL *of* PROSTATE CANCER

First Edition

Up-to-date information about prostate
cancer and therapeutic options

An expert review for the public
and health care practitioners

DR. LUIS MENDOZA

authorHOUSE®

AuthorHouse™ UK Ltd.
500 Avebury Boulevard
Central Milton Keynes, MK9 2BE
www.authorhouse.co.uk
Phone: 08001974150

Published by AuthorHouse 01/04/2013

ISBN: 978-1-4817-8038-4 (sc)

This publication about prostate cancer is part of a continuing public and professional education program. During the last decade the therapeutic spectrum of prostate cancer has changed dramatically. This prostate cancer manual is intended to present the complex nature of this cancer, the standard treatments and new therapeutic alternatives that have recently been approved and bring new possibilities of a cure.

This manual is not intended as a substitute for professional healthcare. It is a preliminary guide to educate patients about treatment options and about the disease itself, so they will be better prepared to discuss it with their health care practitioners.

Due to the high level of the scientific information content, this manual is also for students of medicine and healthcare professionals in general.

CONTENTS

INTRODUCTION

The prostate is a gland found only in males and is an organ forming part of the male reproductive system. It is located immediately below the bladder and just in front of the bowel. Its main function is to produce fluid which protects and enriches sperm. The size of the prostate varies with age. In younger men, it is about the size of a wal-nut, but it can be much larger in older men. The tube that carries urine (the urethra) runs through the center of the prostate. Male hormones (called androgens) such as testosterone cause

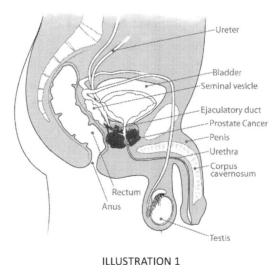

ILLUSTRATION 1

Anatomy of the genitourinary system in a male. The illustration shows a prostate cancer situated in the prostate gland, which is below the bladder.

this growth. The prostate contains cells that make some of the fluid (semen) that protects and nourishes the sperm. The nerves that control erections surround the prostate.

1

Prostate cancer is the most frequent and second most lethal malignancy (cancerous growth) in men. Survival after prostate cancer diagnosis can often exceed a decade and fewer than 5% of men without metastatic disease (cancerous cell growth from an original site to one or more sites elsewhere in the body) at diagnosis will die from prostate cancer within the first 5 to 10 years after diagnosis. Prostate cancer is extremely common, affecting 15% of white men and 18% of African American men throughout their lifetime, and it will result in death in 3% of men in North America. The disease is comparable to breast cancer, which will affect 12% of women throughout their lifetime and cause death in 3%.

Fortunately, the mortality trends for prostate cancer have been declining, and according to some experts, this may suggest that early detection using the prostate-specific antigen (PSA) test or digital rectal exam (DRE) may be beneficial. Since 1994, the rate of death from the disease has been declining by 4.1 percent annually. However, prostate cancer is still the second leading cause of cancer death.

In the USA, the age-adjusted incidence rate (number of diagnosed cases of prostate cancer) is around 154 per 100,000 men per year and the age-adjusted death rate (number of death due to prostate cancer) is around 24 per 100,000 men per year. The last decade has seen huge advances in the understanding of the biology of prostate cancer which has allowed the development of novel agents. Four new treatments of metastatic prostate cancer have been recently approved: sipulleucel-T, denosumab, cabazitaxel and abiraterone acetate and there are several other agents waiting to be approved soon. This manual reviews all prostate cancer treatments which have been approved by the scientific community up to the present time.

PROSTATE CANCER SCREENING

Screening is an important part of the early detection and diagnosis of the prostate cancer. It involves testing for prostate cancer in men with no symptoms of the disease. Initial suspicion of prostate cancer is based on an abnormal DRE or an abnormal test for PSA (prostate specific antigen).

DRE is a medical examination where the physician inserts a lubricated, gloved finger into the rectum to determine if the prostate is harder than normal or is abnormal in size or shape. DRE results can give you and your doctor a great deal of information in a short amount of time. During such exploration the physician will able to determine if the prostate gland is normal or abnormal. The presence of an area of increased hardness, presence of a nodule or bump, overall increase in size and feeling of being tender to the touch are medical findings which confirm that the prostate gland is abnormal.

The abnormalities of the prostate gland can be due to multiple reasons. However, it is important to rule out a diagnosis of prostate cancer. Unfortunately, some men develop prostate cancer without any detectable abnormality in their DRE. Therefore, we can't exclusively rely on a DRE; the PSA test is needed to complete the screening for early detection of the prostate cancer.

The PSA test measures the amount of prostate specific antigen in the blood. PSA is released into a man's blood by his prostate gland. Healthy men have low amounts of PSA in the blood. The amount of PSA in the blood normally increases as a man's prostate enlarges with age. PSA may increase because of inflammation of the prostate gland (prostatitis) or prostate cancer.

A PSA value of 4.0 ng/ml or less is considered normal; however, 15% of men with this "normal" PSA will have prostate cancer and 2% will have high-grade cancer. The results of three large clinical trials designed to determine the effectiveness of PSA testing were inconclusive. Further studies are under way. Most experts agree that the current evidence is insufficient to recommend for or against routine testing for early prostate cancer detection. The American Cancer Society recommends that asymptomatic (in good health without exhibiting symptoms of disease) men who have at least a 10-year life expectancy have an opportunity to make an informed decision with their doctors about whether or not to be screened for prostate cancer after receiving information about the uncertainties, risks and potential benefits associated with PSA.

RISK FACTORS FOR PROSTATE CANCER

There are several major factors that influence risk, some of which unfortunately, cannot be changed.

Age: The older you are, the more likely you are to be diagnosed with prostate cancer. Although only 1 in 10,000 men under the age of 40 will be diagnosed, the rate shoots up to 1 in 38 for ages 40 to 59, and 1 in 15 for ages 60 to 69. In fact, more than 65% of all prostate cancers are diagnosed in men over the age of 65. The average age at diagnosis of prostate cancer in the United States is 69. After that age, the chance of developing prostate cancer becomes more common than any other cancer in men or women.

Race: African American men are 60% more likely to develop prostate cancer compared with Caucasian men and are nearly 2.5 times as likely to die from the disease. Conversely, Asian men who live in Asia have the lowest risk.

Family history/genetics: A man with a father or brother who developed prostate cancer is twice as likely to develop the disease. This risk is further increased if the cancer was diagnosed in family members at a younger age (less than 55 years of age) or if it affected three or more family members.

Geographical location: For men in the U.S., the risk of developing prostate cancer is 17%. For men who live in rural China, it's 2%. However, when Chinese men move to the Western countries, their risk increases substantially.

Men who live in cities north of 40 degrees latitude (north of Philadelphia, PA, Columbus, OH, and Provo, UT, for instance) have the highest risk of dying from prostate cancer of any men in the United States. This effect appears to be mediated by inadequate sunlight during three months of the year, which reduces vitamin D levels.

Body Mass Index (BMI), physical activity and diet: Many prospective studies have consistently demonstrated an increased prostate cancer mortality rate among men with higher BMI but most have not distinguished whether this association is due to an increased risk of having an aggressive disease at the diagnosis or worse outcomes after initial diagnosis. Also many studies found an inverse association between physical activity and prostate cancer risk; however, more studies are needed to be conclusive. There is also an association between consumption of high saturated fat and prostate cancer. Research in the past few years has shown that diet modification might decrease the chances of developing prostate cancer, reduce the likelihood of having a prostate cancer recurrence, or help slow the progression of the disease.

MYTHS ABOUT RISK FACTORS FOR PROSTATE CANCER

Sexual Activity: High levels of sexual activity or frequent ejaculation have been rumored to increase prostate cancer risk. This is untrue. In fact, studies show that men who reported more frequent ejaculations had a lower risk of developing prostate cancer.

Vasectomy: Having a vasectomy was originally thought to increase a man's risk, but this has since been disproven.

Alcohol: There is no link between alcohol and prostate cancer risk.

PROSTATE CANCER PREVENTION

Many prostate cancer risk factors, such as race and genetics, cannot be changed. Men with an increased risk of disease, including African Americans or those with a family history of prostate cancer, may consider following a strategy to reduce the risk. To date, two approaches, chemoprevention, and diet & lifestyle modifications, have been evaluated for preventing prostate cancer.

Chemoprevention: Chemoprevention is defined as the use of specific natural (dietary) or synthetic agents to prevent, delay, or slow down the carcinogenic process. Prostate cancer is an ideal target disease for chemoprevention thanks to long latency, high incidence, availability of reliable test for early cancer detection like the PSA, identifiable preneoplastic (abnormal change in the structure of the cells of the prostate gland before the formation of a cancer) lesions and a large subgroup of good prognosis patients with long survival.

Many potential interventions have been proposed for the prevention of prostate cancer. These interventions include medications (5-α reductase inhibitors, nonsteroidal anti-inflammatory drugs [NSAIDs], Cox 2 inhibitors, selective estrogen receptor modulators [SERMs], statins); dietary supplements (vitamins A, C, D, and E, selenium, calcium, multivitamins, folic acid, lycopene, soy and related isoflavanoids, green tea and related polyphenols, omega 3/6 fatty acids); and dietary interventions (soy, fat, protein, and fish consumption). From the above interventions, 5-α reductase inhibitors are the most extensively studied drugs for the prevention of prostate cancer. However, either dutatsteride or finasteride, which are currently approved to treat benign prostate enlargement, haven't been approved by the FDA for prostate cancer prevention due to the risk of increasing high-grade prostate cancer.

I have to note here, that recent reports suggest that 25-50% of prostate cancer patients use at least one complementary or alternative medicine. The most common of these medicines are vitamin and herbal preparations with purported antitumor effect despite only modest underlying preclinical and clinical evidence of efficacy. From the reviewed available clinical data, experts conclude that there is insufficient evidence to support the use of medicines for the treatment of prostate cancer patients outside of a clinical trial.

Diet and lifestyle modifications: In the meantime, diet and lifestyle modifications have been shown to reduce the risk of prostate cancer development and progression, and can help men with prostate cancer live longer and better lives.

RECOMMENDATIONS FOR PREVENTING PROSTATE CANCER

Given the facts that some prostate cancer risk factors, such as race and genetics are difficult to change, there are still many things that men can do to reduce or delay their risk of developing prostate cancer. Trying to understand why prostate cancer is so common in the West and much less so in Asia, and why, when Asian men migrate to the West the risk of prostate cancer increase over time, experts believe the major factor (which explain it) is diet – foods that produce damage to DNA (deoxyribonucleic acid, the primary carrier of genetic information found in the chromosomes). So what can you do to prevent or delay the onset of the disease?

1. Cut down on your calorie intake or exercise more so that you maintain a healthy weight.
2. Try to keep the amount of fat you get from red meat and dairy products to a minimum. Eat more fish – evidence from studies suggests that fish can help protect against prostate cancer because they contain "good fat", particularly omega-3 fatty acids. Avoid trans fatty acids (found in margarine). Try to incorporate cooked tomatoes that are cooked with olive oil, which has also been shown to be beneficial and cruciferous vegetables (like broccoli and cauliflower) into many of your weekly meals. Soy and green tea are also potential dietary components that may be helpful.

11

3. Avoid over-supplementation with megavitamins. While a multivitamin is not likely to be harmful, if you follow a healthy diet with plenty of fruits, vegetables, whole grains, fish, and healthy oils, you probably don't need to take multivitamins. Do not take supplements far above the recommended daily allowance. New evidence about the effect of vitamin E on prostate cancer risk may make some men think twice before they pop a daily supplement. Researchers at the National Cancer Institute found that men who took a high daily dose of vitamin E had a 17 percent greater risk of developing prostate cancer.

4. Avoid smoking for many reasons. Alcohol in moderation, if at all.

5. Seek medical treatment for stress, high blood pressure, high cholesterol, and depression. Treating these conditions may save your life and will improve your chances of survival.

DIAGNOSIS

As soon as your physician has found an abnormal prostate (presence of a nodule/s or a change in its consistency) and/or an abnormal PSA, you will be given a thorough examination to confirm or exclude a diagnosis of prostate cancer.

Symptoms: Not everyone experiences symptoms of prostate cancer. In many cases, signs of prostate cancer are first detected by a doctor during a routine check-up. Some men, however, will experience changes in urinary or sexual function that might indicate the presence of prostate cancer. These symptoms include:

- A need to urinate frequently, especially at night

- Difficulty starting urination or holding back urine

- Weak or interrupted flow of urine

- Painful or burning urination

- Difficulty in having an erection

- Painful ejaculation

- Blood in urine or semen

- Frequent pain or stiffness in the lower back, hips, or upper thighs

Please note that these symptoms can also indicate the presence of other diseases or disorders of the prostate, such as benign prostate hypertrophy (BPH) (enlargement of the prostate) or prostatitis (inflammation of the prostate).

Prostate Specific Antigen (PSA): Prostate specific antigen, or PSA, is a protein produced by cells of the prostate gland. The PSA test measures the level of PSA in a man's blood. For this test, a blood sample is sent to a laboratory for analysis. The results are usually reported as nanograms of PSA per millitier (ng/mL) of blood. The blood level of PSA is often higher in men with prostate cancer. In addition to prostate cancer, a number of benign (not cancerous) conditions can cause a man's PSA level to rise. The most frequent benign prostate conditions that cause an increase in PSA level are prostatitis and BPH. There is no evidence that prostatitis or BPH leads to prostate cancer, but it is possible for a man to have one or both of these conditions and to develop prostate cancer as well.

Interpretation of PSA test results

There is no specific normal or abnormal level of PSA in the blood. In the past, most doctors considered PSA levels of 4.0 ng/mL and lower as normal. Therefore, if a man had a PSA level above 4.0 ng/mL, doctors would often recommend a prostate biopsy (see section "Prostate Biopsy") to determine whether prostate cancer was present. However, more recent studies have shown that some men with PSA levels below 4.0 ng/mL have prostate cancer and that many men with higher levels do not have prostate cancer. Another complicating factor is that studies to establish the normal range of PSA levels have been conducted primarily in populations of white men.

Although expert opinions vary, there is no clear consensus regarding the optimal PSA threshold for recommending a prostate biopsy for men of any racial or ethnic group. In general, however, the higher a man's PSA level, the more likely it is that he has prostate cancer. Moreover, a continuous rise in a man's PSA level over time may also be a sign of prostate cancer.

Following PSA levels during and after treatment

The PSA level is often a good indicator of how effective treatment is or has been. Generally speaking, your PSA level should reach levels below 4.0 ng/mL after treatment. After surgery the PSA should fall to an undetectable level within a couple of months after radical prostatectomy (surgical removal of the prostate gland). After radiation therapy the pattern of the drop in PSA is also different from after surgery. PSA levels after radiation tend to drop gradually, and may not reach their lowest level until 2 years or more after treatment.

During hormone therapy, chemotherapy, or vaccine therapy, these treatments are used for more advanced prostate cancer and the PSA level can help indicate how well the treatment is working or when it may be time to try a different form of treatment. Treatments should lower the PSA level (at least at first), although in some cases they may just help keep it from rising further, or even just slow the rise. Before starting anticancer treatment, you might want to ask your doctor what he or she expects your PSA level to be during and after treatment, and what levels might be worrying. It's also important to know that PSA levels may fluctuate a bit on their own in some cases. Many men being treated for prostate cancer are very concerned about even the smallest of changes in their PSA levels.

The blood PSA level is an important tool to monitor the cancer, but not every rise in PSA necessarily means that the cancer is growing and requires treatment right away. To help avoid unnecessary anxiety, be sure you understand what level of change in PSA your doctor might consider to be a cause for concern.

During active surveillance

If you choose active surveillance (See the section "active surveillance" for more details.), your PSA level will be monitored closely (most likely along with other tests) to help decide whether the cancer is growing and if other types of treatment should be considered.

PROSTATE BIOPSY

If certain symptoms or the results of early detection tests – a PSA blood test and/or DRE – suggest that you might have prostate cancer, your doctor will do a prostate biopsy to find out.

A biopsy is a procedure in which a sample of body tissue is removed and then looked at under a microscope. A core needle biopsy is the main method used to diagnose prostate cancer. It is usually done by a urologist, a surgeon who treats cancers of the genital and urinary tract, which includes the prostate gland.

To perform the biopsy, the urologist uses the transrectal ultrasound. It generates sound waves to make an image of the prostate on a video screen. For this test, a small probe that gives off sound waves is placed into the rectum. The sound waves enter the prostate and create echoes that are picked up by the probe. A computer turns the pattern of echoes into a black and white image of the prostate. Using transrectal ultrasound to "see" the prostate gland, the doctor quickly inserts a thin, hollow needle through the wall of the rectum into the prostate gland. When the needle is pulled out it removes a small cylinder (core) of prostate tissue. This is repeated from 8 to 18 times, but most urologists will take about 12 samples.

Though the procedure sounds painful, it usually causes only a brief uncomfortable sensation. Most doctors who do the biopsy will numb the area first by injecting a local anesthetic alongside the prostate. The biopsy itself takes about 10 minutes and is usually done in the doctor's office. You will

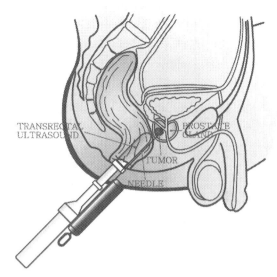

ILLUSTRATION 2

Transrectal ultrasound guided biopsy of a tumor situated in the prostate, using a needle.

likely be given antibiotics to take before the biopsy and possibly for a day or 2 after to reduce the risk of infection.

For a few days after the procedure, you may feel some soreness in the area and will probably notice blood in your urine. You may also have some light bleeding from your rectum, especially if you have hemorrhoids. Many men also see some blood in their semen or have rust colored semen, which can last for several weeks after the biopsy, depending on how frequently you ejaculate.

Your biopsy samples will be sent to a lab, where a pathologist (a doctor who specializes in diagnosing disease in tissue samples) will look at them under a microscope to see if they contain cancer cells. If cancer is present, the pathologist will also assign it a grade (see the next section). Getting the results usually takes at least 1 to 3 days, but it can take longer.

Even taking many samples, biopsies can still sometimes miss a cancer if none of the biopsy needles pass through it. This is known as a "false negative" result. If your doctor still strongly suspects you have prostate cancer (due to a very high PSA level, for example) a repeat biopsy may be needed to help to be sure.

REPORT FROM THE BIOPSY

A doctor typically diagnoses prostate cancer after closely examining biopsy cells through a microscope. There are several types of cells in the prostate, and each contributes in its own way to the prostate's development, architecture, and function.

Cancer cells look different than normal prostate cells. Pathologists look for the differences, first to detect the presence of cancer and then to determine the grade of cancer malignity.

Gleason Grading

The Gleason grading is the most utilized method to assess the grading of the prostate cancer. The Gleason grading system accounts for the five distinct patterns that prostate tumor cells tend to go through as they change from normal cells to tumor cells.

The cells are scored on a scale from 1 to 5:

- **"Low-grade" tumor cells** (those closest to 1) tend to look very similar to normal cells.

- **"High-grade" tumor cells** (closest to 5) have mutated so much that they often barely resemble the normal cells.

- **Tumor cells grades 2 through 4** have features in between these extremes.

The pathologist looking at the biopsy sample assigns one Gleason grade to the most similar pattern in your biopsy and a second Gleason grade to the second most similar pattern. The Gleason score (between 2 and 10) is determined by adding the Gleason grade of the two most predominant samples of the pathological specimen. Generally speaking, cancers with lower Gleason scores (2 - 4) tend to be less aggressive, while cancers with higher Gleason scores (7 – 10) tend to be more aggressive.

PROSTATE CANCER STAGING

Prostate cancer grows locally within the prostate, often for many years. Eventually, prostate cancer extends outside the prostate. Prostate cancer can spread beyond the prostate in three ways:

- By growing into neighboring tissues (invasion)

- By spreading through the lymph system of lymph nodes and lymph vessels

- By traveling to distant tissues through the blood (metastasis)

After a prostate cancer diagnosis, tests are done to detect how the cancer has spread, if at all, outside the prostate. Not all men need every test. It depends on the characteristics of a man's prostate cancer detected by a biopsy and other clinical factors. Tests to help determine the extension of the disease and subsequently stage of prostate cancer include:

- DRE

- PSA (blood test)

- Transrectal ultrasound

- MRI (magnetic resonance imaging) of the prostate

- CT (computed tomography) scan of the abdomen and pelvis, looking for prostate cancer metastasis to other organs

- Nuclear medicine bone scan, to look for metastasis to bones

- Histological examination of the specimen to examine the prostate cancer spread in lymph nodes of the pelvis

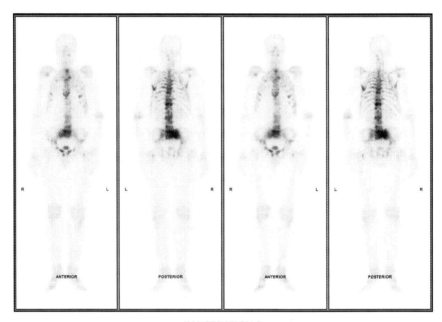

ILLUSTRATION 3

The bone scan shows many dark dots in the spine and ribs which represent the dissemination of the prostate cancer to the bones. Courtesy of Dr. Agnieszka Warszewska.

The stage is based on the prostate biopsy results (including the Gleason score), the PSA level, and any other exams or tests that were done to find out how far the cancer has spread.

The TNM System for Prostate Cancer Stages

As they do for most cancers, doctors use the TNM system of prostate cancer stages. Prostate cancer stages are described using three different aspects of tumor growth and spread. It's called the TNM system for tumor (T), lymph nodes (N), and metastasis (M):

- T - for primary (local) tumor - describes the local extension of the prostate cancer in the prostatic gland.

- N - for lymph nodes - describes whether prostate cancer has spread to any lymph nodes.

- M - for metastasis - means distant spread of prostate cancer, for example, to the bones or liver.

There are 4 categories for describing the local extent of a prostate tumor, ranging from T1 to T4. Most of these have subcategories as well.

T1: Your doctor can't feel the tumor or see it with imaging such as transrectal ultrasound.

- **T1a:** Cancer is found incidentally (by accident) during a transurethral resection of the prostate (TURP), which is a surgical removal of a portion of the prostate through the urethra, that was done for benign prostatic hyperplasia BPH). Cancer is in no more than 5% of the tissue removed.

- **T1b:** Cancer is found during a TURP but is in more than 5% of the tissue removed.

- **T1c:** Cancer is found by needle biopsy that was done because of an increased PSA.

T2: Your doctor can feel the cancer with a DRE or see it with imaging such as transrectal ultrasound, but it still appears to be confined to the prostate gland.

- **T2a:** The cancer is in one half or less of only one side (left or right) of your prostate.

- **T2b:** The cancer is in more than half of only one side (left or right) of your prostate.

- **T2c:** The cancer is in both sides of your prostate.

T3: The cancer has begun to grow and spread outside your prostate and may have spread into the seminal vesicles.

- **T3a:** The cancer extends outside the prostate but not to the seminal vesicles (see figure 1).

- **T3b:** The cancer has spread to the seminal vesicles.

T4: The cancer has grown into tissues next to your prostate (other than the seminal vesicles), such as the urethral sphincter (muscle that helps control urination), the rectum, the bladder, and/or the wall of the pelvis.

N
- N0 (N zero) means that the cancer has not spread to any lymph nodes.

- N1 means the cancer has spread to one or more regional lymph nodes (near the prostate) of the pelvis.

M
- M0 (M zero) means the cancer has no distant metastases.

- M1 means the cancer has spread to nearby (outside the pelvis), and other lymph nodes (such as periaortic or mediastinal), other organs such as bone, lung, liver or brain.

Once the T, N and M, have been determined this information is combined with the Gleason score in a process called group stage. Most stadiums are named in Roman numerals from I (the least advanced) to IV (the most advanced). This is to determine treatment and prognosis. This is a fairly common that doctors set the stage prostate cancer as discussed below

Prostate Cancer Stage I

In stage I, prostate cancer is found in the prostate only. Stage I prostate cancer is microscopic; it can't be felt on a digital rectal exam (DRE), and it isn't seen on imaging of the prostate.

Prostate Cancer Stage II

In stage II, the tumor has grown inside the prostate but hasn't extended beyond it. Possible combinations of the TNM system to stage II are:

- T1a, N0, M0, Gleason intermediate or high (5 to 10)

- T1b, N0, M0, any Gleason (2-10)

- T1c, N0, M0, any Gleason (2-10)

- T2, N0, M0, any Gleason (2-10)

Prostate Cancer Stage III

Stage III prostate cancer has spread outside the prostate, but only barely. Prostate cancer in stage III may involve nearby tissues, like the seminal vesicles.

- T3, N0, M0, any Gleason (2-10)

Prostate Cancer Stage IV

In stage IV, the cancer has spread (metastasized) outside the prostate to other tissues. Stage IV prostate cancer commonly spreads to the bones, lymph nodes, liver, or lungs. Possible combinations of the TNM system to stage IV are:

- T4, N0, M0, any Gleason (2-10)

- Any T, N1, M0, any Gleason (2-10)

- Any T, any N, M1, any Gleason (2-10)

Accurately identifying the prostate cancer stage is extremely important. Prostate cancer stage helps determine the optimal treatment, as well as prognosis. For this reason, it's worth going through extensive testing to get the correct prostate cancer stage.

NOMOGRAMS AND PREDICTIVE MODELS

An optimal treatment approach of prostate cancer always requires evaluation the risk of cancer spread that may not be visible. Therefore, it is important that the health care practitioner assesses on a case-by-case basis risks such as how likely is a given cancer to be confined to the prostate or to spread to regional nodules? or how likely is the cancer to progress or metastasize after treatment? or how likely is salvage or rescue by adjuvant radiation therapy (treatment of the disease by means of ionizing radiation) after an unsuccessful radical prostatectomy (surgical removal of the prostate)? Predicting prognosis is essential for patient decision-making, treatment selection, and adjuvant therapy.

You may have heard your doctor talk about certain tables and nomograms (graphical representation of a statistical model containing scales for calculating the prognostic weight of a value for each individual variable), which are used to predict prostate cancer behavior. Tables and nomograms are characterized by clinical stage of prostate cancer patients determined by DRE, serum PSA levels, Gleason score and imaging studies (Ultrasound, bone scan etc).

Partin tables were the first prediction method used to predict whether the tumor will be confined to the prostate. The tables are based on the accumulated experience of urologists performing radical prostatectomy. D'Amico tables provide predictive information on PSA recurrence for patients treated with radical prostatectomy and radiation therapy. D'Amico and colleagues first proposed a three-group risk stratification system to predict post-treatment biochemical failure (PSA remaining high) after radical prostatectomy and external-beam radiotherapy: (1) low –T1-T2a, PSA ≤10 ng/mL and Gleason ≤6; (2) intermediate –T1-T2, PSA ≤20 ng/mL and Gleason ≤7 not otherwise low-risk; and (3) high-risk –T3-T4 or PSA >20 ng/mL or Gleason 8–10).

To quantify risk more accurately, one can devise a nomogram that incorporates the interactive effects of multiple prognostic factors to make more accurate predictions about the stage and prognosis for the individual patient. With nomograms, discordant values (e.g. high PSA but low Gleason score and clinical stage) can be incorporated into a more accurate prediction. None of the current models predict with perfect accuracy, and only some of these models predict metastasis and cancer-specific death. New independent prognostic factors, using molecular markers and other radiologic evaluations of the prostate, are being developed. These new approaches remain investigational and are not available to or confirmed by the current medical practice. If you are interested in calculating the risks of your prostate cancer yourself I recommend visiting the following web page:

http://nomograms.mskcc.org/Prostate/index.aspx

TREATMENT OPTIONS FOR LOCALIZED PROSTATE CANCER

Treatment options for localized prostate cancer, stage I, include active surveillance, surgery and radiation therapy. There is no consensus about what it is the best local treatment for localized prostate cancer. By discussing your options with your doctor, you can determine the approach that will be best for you.

Active surveillance

Active surveillance (also referred to as observation or watchful waiting) is often used to mean monitoring the cancer closely with PSA blood tests, DRE exams, and ultrasounds at regular intervals to see if the cancer is growing. Clinicians only offer active surveillance to patients whose prostate cancers are at low risk of progressing to life-threatening disease. If there is a change in your test results, your doctor will then talk to you about treatment options. Some men are not comfortable with this approach, and are willing to accept the possible side effects of active treatments in order to try to remove or destroy the cancer.

With active surveillance, your cancer will be carefully monitored. Usually this approach includes a doctor's visit with a PSA blood test and DRE about every 6 months. Transrectal ultrasound-guided prostate biopsies may be done every year as well. Active treatment, either surgery or radiation therapy, can be started if the cancer seems to be growing or getting worse, based on a rising PSA level or a change in the DRE, ultrasound findings, or biopsy results.

Ultimately, a recommendation for active surveillance must be based on a carefully individualized weighing of a number of factors: life expectancy, disease characteristics, general health condition, potential side effects of treatment, and patient preference.

SURGERY

Surgery is a common choice to try to cure prostate cancer if it is not thought to have spread outside the gland (stage I cancers). The main type of surgery for prostate cancer is known as a radical prostatectomy. In this operation, the surgeon removes the entire prostate gland plus some of the tissue around it, including the seminal vesicles. However, because of the morbidity (potential perioperative complications), radical prostatectomy should be reserved for patients whose life expectancy is 10 years or more.

There are different ways to perform a radical prostatectomy: radical retropubic prostatectomy, radical perineal prostatectomy, laparoscopic radical prostatectomy and Robotic-assisted laparoscopic radical prostatectomy (see below).

Radical retropubic prostatectomy

For this operation, the surgeon makes a skin incision in your lower abdomen, from the belly button down to the pubic bone. You will be either under general anesthesia (asleep) or be given spinal or epidural anesthesia (numbing the lower half of the body) along with sedation during the surgery.

If there is a reasonable chance the cancer may have spread to the lymph nodes (based on your PSA level, DRE, and biopsy results), the surgeon first may remove lymph nodes from around the prostate at this time. The nodes are usually sent to the pathology lab to see if they have cancer cells (it takes a few days to get the results), but in some cases the nodes may be looked at right away. If this is done during surgery and any of the nodes have cancer cells, which means the cancer has spread, the surgeon may not continue with the surgery. This is because it is unlikely that the cancer can be cured with surgery, and removing the prostate could still lead to serious side effects.

If the surgeon decides to continue with removing the prostate, he/she will pay close attention to the 2 tiny bundles of nerves that run on either side of the prostate. These nerves control erections. If you are able to have erections before surgery, the surgeon will try not to injure these nerves (known as a nerve-sparing approach). If the cancer is growing into or very close to the nerves the surgeon will need to remove them. If they are both removed, you will be unable to have spontaneous erections. This means that you will need help (such as medicines or pumps) to have erections. If the nerves on one side are removed, you still have a chance of keeping your ability to have erections, but the chance is lower than if neither were removed. If neither nerve bundle is removed you may be able to function normally. Usually it takes at least a few months to a year after surgery to have an erection because the nerves have been handled during the operation and won't work properly for a while.

Radical perineal prostatectomy

In this operation, the surgeon makes the incision in the skin between the anus and scrotum, in a region called the perineum. This approach is used less often because the nerves cannot easily be spared and lymph nodes can't be removed. But it is often a shorter operation and might be an option if you don't want the nerve-sparing procedure and you don't require lymph node removal, and is often easier to recover from. It might also be used if you have other medical conditions that make retropubic surgery difficult for you. It can be just as curative as the retropubic approach if done correctly. The perineal operation usually takes less time than the retropubic operation, and may result in less pain afterward.

Laparoscopic radical prostatectomy

For a laparoscopic radical prostatectomy, the surgeon makes several small incisions, through which the laparoscope, which is a flexible illuminated fiberoptic instrument, is inserted through the belly to remove the prostate. The laparoscope has a small video camera on the end, which lets the surgeon see inside the abdomen. LRP has been used in the United States since 1999. Early studies report that the rates of side effects from LRP seem to be about the same as for traditional radical prostatectomies.

Laparoscopic prostatectomy has some advantages over the usual open radical prostatectomy, including less blood loss and pain, shorter hospital stays (usually no more than a day), and faster recovery times (although a catheter will be needed for about the same amount of time).

Robotic-assisted laparoscopic radical prostatectomy

A newer approach is to do the laparoscopic surgery remotely using a robotic interface (called the da Vinci system), which is known as robotic-assisted laparoscopic prostatectomy (RALRP). The surgeon sits at a panel near the operating table and controls robotic arms to perform the operation through several small incisions in the patient's abdomen.

Like direct LRP, RALRP has advantages in terms of less pain, blood loss, and recovery time. So far though, there seems to be little difference in efficacy between robotic and direct LRP for the patient.

In terms of the side effects men are most concerned about, such as urinary problems or erectile dysfunction (described below), there does not seem to be a difference between robotic-assisted LRP and other approaches to prostatectomy.

Robotic LRP has been in use since 2003 in the United States and is now the most common way to do a prostatectomy.

If you decide that either type of LRP is the treatment for you, be sure to find a surgeon with a lot of experience. Again,

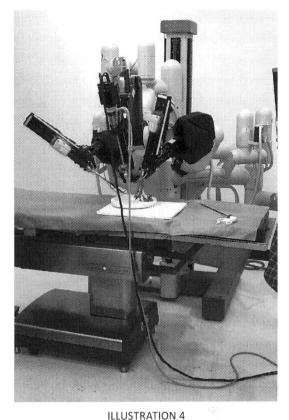

ILLUSTRATION 4

Surgery bed showing the arms of the robot (Da Vinci system) to perform radical prostatectomies in patients with localized prostate cancer.

the most important factors for a successful treatment are likely to be the skill and experience of your surgeon.

Side effects

The major possible side effects of radical prostatectomy are urinary incontinence (being unable to control urine) and impotence (being unable to have erections). It should be noted that these side effects can also occur with other forms of treatment for prostate cancer, although they are described here in more detail.

Urinary incontinence: You may develop urinary incontinence, which means you are not able to control your urine or have leakage or dribbling.

After surgery for prostate cancer, normal bladder control usually returns within several weeks or months. This recovery usually occurs gradually, in stages.

Doctors can't predict for sure how any patient will be affected after surgery. In general older men tend to have more incontinence problems than younger men

Treatment of incontinence depends on its type, cause, and severity. If you have problems with incontinence, let your doctors know. You might feel embarrassed about discussing this issue, but remember that you are not alone. This is a common problem. Doctors who treat men with prostate cancer should know about incontinence and be able to suggest ways to improve it, such as: 1) special exercises, called Kegel exercises; *2)* medicines and 3) surgery using collagen to tighten the bladder sphincter or implanting an artificial sphincter. Ask your doctor if these treatments might help you.

Even if your incontinence cannot completely be corrected, it can still be helped. You can learn how to manage and live with incontinence. Incontinence is more than a physical problem. It can disrupt your quality of life if it is not managed well. There is no one right way to cope with incontinence. The challenge is to find what works for you so that you can return to your normal daily activities.

There are many incontinence products that can help keep you mobile and comfortable, such as pads that are worn under your clothing. Another option is a rubber sheath called a condom catheter that can be put over the penis to collect urine in a bag. There are also compression (pressure) devices – penile clamps- that can be placed on the penis for short periods of time to help keep urine from coming out. For some types of incontinence, self-catheterization with urethral inserts may be an option. In this approach, you insert a thin tube into your urethra to drain and empty the bladder at regular intervals. Most men can learn this safe and usually painless technique.

You can also follow some simple precautions that may make incontinence less of a problem. For example, empty your bladder before bedtime or before strenuous activity. Avoid drinking too much fluid, particularly if the drinks contain caffeine or alcohol, which can make you have to go more often. Fear, anxiety, and anger are common feelings for people dealing with incontinence. Fear of having an accident may keep you from doing the things you enjoy most – taking your grandchild to the park, going to the movies, or playing a round of golf. You may feel isolated and embarrassed. You may even avoid sex because you are afraid of leakage. Be sure to talk to your doctor so you can begin to manage this problem, as many solutions, described above, exist.

Impotence (erectile dysfunction): This means you cannot get an erection sufficient for sexual penetration. The nerves that allow men to get erections may be damaged or removed by radical prostatectomy. Your ability to have an erection after surgery depends on your age, your ability to get an erection before the operation, and whether the nerves were cut. Everyone can expect some decrease in the ability to have an erection after the radical prostatectomy, but the younger you are, the more likely it is that you will keep this ability.

A wide range of impotency rates have been reported in the medical literature, from as low as about 1 in 4 men under age 60 to as high as about 3 in 4 men over age 70. Surgeons with large experience of performing a nerve-sparing radical prostatectomies tend to report lower impotence rates.

Each man's situation is different, so the best way to get an idea of your chances for recovering erections is to ask your doctor about his or her success rates and what the outcome is likely to be in your particular case.

If your ability to have erections does return after surgery, it often occurs slowly. In fact, it can take up to 2 years. During the first several months, you will probably not be able to have a spontaneous erection, so you may need to use medicines or other treatments.

If potency remains after surgery, the sensation of orgasm should continue to be pleasurable, but there is no ejaculation of semen – the orgasm is "dry." This is because during the prostatectomy, the glands that made most of the fluid for semen (the seminal vesicles and prostate) were removed, and the pathways used by sperm (the vas deferens) were cut.

Most doctors feel that regaining potency is helped along by attempting to get an erection as soon as possible once the body has had a chance to heal (usually several weeks after the operation). Some doctors call this penile rehabilitation. Medicines (see below) may be helpful at this time. Be sure to talk to your doctor about your situation.

Several options may help you if you have erectile dysfunction: 1) Phosphodiesterase inhibitors such as sildenafil (Viagra), vardenafil (Levitra), and tadalafil (Cialis) are pills that can promote erections. These drugs will not work if both nerves that control erections have been damaged or removed; 2) Alprostadil is a man-made version of prostaglandin E1, a substance naturally made in the body that can produce erections. It can be injected almost painlessly into the base of the penis 5 to 10 minutes before intercourse or placed into the tip of the penis as suppository; 3) Vacuum devices are another option that may create an erection. These mechanical pumps are placed around the entire penis before intercourse to produce an erection and 4) Penile implants might restore your ability to have erections if other methods do not help. There are several types of penile implants, including those using silicone rods or inflatable devices. An operation is needed to put them in place.

RADIATION THERAPY

The goal of radiation therapy for men with localized prostate cancer is to deliver a therapeutic dose of ionizing rays to kill cancer cells. Cure rates for men with these types of cancers are about the same as those for men getting radical prostatectomy. Two main types of radiation therapy can be used: external beam radiation and brachytherapy (internal radiation).

External beam radiation therapy (EBRT)

EBRT, which is the most common type of radiation therapy, the beams of radiation are focused on the prostate gland from a machine outside the body. This type of therapy requires a coordinated care team of radiotherapists including an oncologist, an expert team in radiation, a nurse and a physicist. Together, the specialized equipment and experienced team prescribe, plan, manage and monitor the radiation treatments.

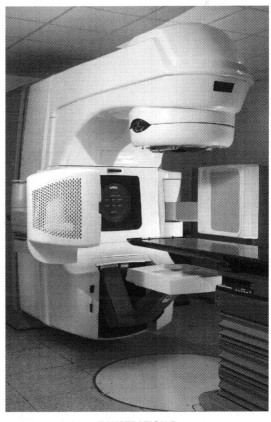

ILLUSTRATION 5

Latest generation irradiation machine, linear accelerator, used for external bean radiation therapy to treat localized prostate cancer.

Over the past several decades, a radiation therapy technique has evolved to allow higher dose of radiation to be administered safely. For example, standard 2-dimensional planning techniques used until the early 1990s limited total doses to 60 – 70 Gy (gray, unit for radiation) due to acute and chronic toxicities. Nowadays physicians use a 3-dimensional (3 D) conformal radiation therapy, which is a technique by which the tumor is targeted from several angles, so the organs in the vicinity of the prostate receive less irradiation. The 3 D radiation therapy uses computer software to integrate CT scan images of the patient's internal anatomy. Newer techniques let doctors give higher doses of radiation to the prostate gland while reducing the radiation exposure to nearby healthy tissues. The 3 D technique provokes fewer side effects.

The results of randomized trials suggested that dose escalation is associated with low tumor recurrences. In light of the new results, the conventional 70 Gy is no longer considered adequate. A dose of 75.6 – 79.2 Gy in conventional fractions to the prostate is appropriate for patients with low-risk cancers. Intermediate-risk and high-risk patients should receive doses up to 81 Gy. Your normal life-style can be maintained during the treatment. The therapy requires a brief daily visit to a treatment center, usually Monday to Friday, for around 2 months.

Possible side effects of EBRT

Thanks to the new radiotherapy techniques undesirable side effects are currently lower than those observed in the past, but even these can be presented. These are:

Bowel problems: During and after treatment with EBRT, you may have diarrhea, sometimes with blood in the stool, rectal leakage, and an irritated large intestine. Most of these problems go away over time, but in rare cases normal bowel function does not return after treatment ends. In the past, about 10% to 20% of men reported bowel problems after

EBRT, but the newer radiation techniques may be less likely to cause these problems.

Bladder problems: You might need to urinate more often, have a burning sensation while you urinate, and/or find blood in your urine. Bladder problems usually improve over time, but in some men they never go away. About 1 in 3 men continues to need to urinate more often after the radiation therapy of the prostate.

Urinary incontinence: Overall, this side effect is less common than after radical prostatectomy, but the chance of incontinence goes up each year for several years after treatment.

Erection problems, including impotence: After a few years, the impotence rate after radiation is about the same as that after radical prostatectomy. It usually does not occur right after radiation therapy but slowly develops over a year or more. This is different from surgery, where impotence occurs immediately and may improve over time. In older studies, about 3 out of 4 men were impotent within 5 years of having EBRT, but some of these men had erection problems before treatment. About half of the men who had normal erections before treatment became impotent after 5 years. It's not clear if these numbers will apply to newer forms of radiation as well.

Feeling tired: Radiation therapy may cause fatigue that may not go away until a few months after treatment stops.

Lymphedema: Fluid buildup in the legs or genitals is possible if the lymph nodes receive radiation.

Urethral stricture: The urethra, which is the conduct that carries urine from the bladder out of the body may, rarely, be scarred and narrowed by radiation. This can cause problems with urination, and may require further treatment to open it up again (dilatation).

Secondary cancers: there is a small increase in the risk of secondary cancers of the bladder and rectum in patients who have had EBRT for prostate cancer. Patients treated with EBRT should be screened regularly for early detection of these cancers.

Brachytherapy (internal radiation therapy)

Brachytherapy (also called *seed implants*) uses small radioactive pellets, or "seeds," each about the size of a grain of rice. These pellets are placed directly into your prostate. There are two types of brachytherapy . Permanent implants (seeds) are used often, while temporary implants emitting higher-dose radiation are employed less frequently. In both cases, because the radioactivity remains inside the prostate, it can be stronger than EBRT, better focused, and constant. In this approach, pellets (seeds) of radioactive material (such as iodine-125 or palladium-103) are placed inside thin needles, which are inserted through the skin in the area between the scrotum and anus and into the prostate. The pellets are left in place as the needles are removed and give off low doses of radiation for weeks or months. Usually, anywhere from 40 to 100 seeds are placed. Ultrasonic devices are used to guide the placements of the seeds in the prostate.

Prostate brachytherapy as monotherapy (as the only given treatment) has become a popular treatment option for early, clinically organ-confined prostate cancer with a Gleason grade 2-6 and PSA < 10 ng/ml. For patients with intermediate-risk cancers, brachytherapy may be combined with ERBT (45 Gy) with or without adjuvant hormone therapy, but the complication rates increase. Patients with high-risk cancers are generally considered poor candidates for permanent brachytherapy; however, with the addition of EBRT and hormone therapy, brachytherapy may be effective in selected patients. The advantage of brachytherapy is that the treatment is completed in 1 day with little time lost from normal activities.

The risk of incontinence is minimal in patients without a previous resection of prostate and the erectile function is preserved. Brachytherapy may not be as effective in men with large prostate glands because it may not be possible to place the seeds into all of the correct locations. Doctors are now looking at ways to get around this, such as giving men a short course of hormone therapy beforehand to shrink the prostate. Disadvantages of brachytherapy include the requirement for general anesthesia and the risk of acute urinary retention. Frequently, discomfort during voiding of urine may persist for as long as 1 year after implantation. During the first two weeks, there is a slight risk of losing one or more seeds during sex or urination. If a seed is lost through urine, you should make sure it is flushed away. Use a condom every time you have sex. You should not have children on your lap for long periods. If so, the maximum time should be one and a half hours per day, for a month and a half.

TREATMENT OPTIONS FOR RECURRENT PROSTATE CANCER

About 30 percent of men treated for localized disease experience a recurrence of prostate cancer. In general, the first manifestation of recurrent prostate cancer is called "biochemical recurrence", which is characterized by a rise in serum PSA levels and normal testosterone levels. When your PSA rises but your testosterone levels are normal it is more likely to reflect prostate cancer recurrence. For patients who have an increase of PSA equal or higher than 0.2 ng / ml PSA after radical prostatectomy and for patients with an increase of PSA of 2 ng/ml or more above the lowest level reached after treatment after radiation therapy may be worrying and might indicate recurrence. Some doctors suggest monitoring PSA levels and others a complementary treatment. If it is observed by monitoring the increase of PSA, then a recurrence of the cancer is confirmed and a complementary treatment should be started. Most patients with recurrent prostate cancer PSA have an increase without symptoms.

Treatment of recurrent prostate cancer may include the following, depending on whether the disease is still considered local (recurrence only at the prostate gland) or disseminated when the disease has disseminated to other parts of the body. The recommendations are the following:

1. For local recurrence the local salvage therapies with surgery or radiation therapy after failure of radiation therapy and prostatectomy, respectively is used. Other surgical alternatives like ultrasound-guided cryosurgery (freezing of prostate cancer cells) or high-intensity focused ultrasound therapy (HIFU) using heat delivered through ultrasound energy to destroy cancer cells has been approved in some countries

2. For various stages of the disease (localized and disseminated) androgen-deprivation therapy (ADT) is used

3. For disseminated recurrence biologic therapy and chemotherapy are used. Drugs for treatment of bone metastasis and radioisotopes such as strontium-89 are also used in clinical practice

ANDROGEN-DEPRIVATION THERAPY (ADT)

Androgen deprivation therapy (ADT) is also called hormone therapy or androgen suppression therapy. The goal is to reduce levels of male hormones, called androgens, in the body, or to prevent them from reaching prostate cancer cells. The main androgens are testosterone and dihydrotestosterone (DHT). Androgens, which are made mainly in the testicles, stimulate prostate cancer cells to grow. Lowering androgen levels or stopping them from getting into prostate cancer cells often makes prostate cancers shrink or grow more slowly for a time. However, hormone therapy alone does not cure prostate cancer when it has grown beyond the prostate gland.

ADT is commonly used in the treatment of prostate cancer. Several types of ADT can be used to treat prostate cancer: bilateral orchiectomy (surgical castration) or a luteinizing-hormone releasing hormone (LHRH, also know gonadotropin-releasing hormone or GnRH) agonists (also called analogs) or LHRH antagonist (see below). Response to hormone therapy can be measured by decline in PSA values, decrease in the size of nodal or visceral metastases, or improvement in cancer-related symptoms. Overall, 60% to

70% of patients with abnormal PSA levels will have normalization of the PSA to below 4 ng/ml after castration, 30% to 50% of determined tumor metastasis will regress by 50% or more of their sizes, and 60% of patients see an improvement in their urinary symptoms and pain.

Bilateral orchiectomy (surgical castration)

Even though this is a type of surgery, its main effect is as a form of hormone therapy. In this operation, the surgeon removes the testicles, where most of the androgens (testosterone and DHT) are made. With this source removed, most prostate cancers stop growing or shrink for a time. This is done as a simple outpatient procedure. It is probably the least expensive and simplest way to reduce androgen levels in the body and to treat a disseminated prostate cancer. But unlike some of the other methods of lowering androgen levels, it is permanent, and many men have trouble accepting the removal of their testicles despite there being an acceptable cosmetic replacement by testicles of silicone.

LHRH agonists

These drugs lower the amount of testosterone made by the testicles. Even though LHRH agonists (or analogs) cost more than bilateral orchiectomy and require more frequent doctor visits, most men choose this method. These drugs allow the testicles to remain in place; however, patients should be aware that the testicles shrink over time. LHRH agonists are injected or placed as small implants under the skin. The LHRH analogs approved include leuprolide (Lupron®, Viadur®, Eligard®), goserelin (Zoladex®), triptorelin (Trelstar®), and histrelin (Vantas®).

When LHRH analogs are first given, testosterone levels go up briefly before falling to very low levels. This effect is called flare. Flare is an inflammatory reaction in the metastasis and sometimes misinterpreted as cancer growth. Men whose cancer has spread to the bones may experience pain in their bones or a worsening of the pain with LHRH agonists. The patient may experience a compression of the spinal cord which can cause pain or paralysis. Flare can be avoided by giving anti-androgens therapy (see below) at least 7 days before starting treatment with LHRH agonists.

LHRH antagonists

Unlike LHRH agonists, LHRH antagonists rapidly reduce testosterone and do not cause tumor flare. Degarelix (Firmagon®) is the first LHRH antagonist approved by the Food and Drug Administration (FDA) in 2008 for treatment of advanced prostate cancer. Ninety six percent of patients receiving degarelix had testosterone ≤ 50 ng/ml within 3 days. It is given as a monthly injection under the skin and achieves the same level of testosterone suppression as leuprolide. However, due to its site of subcutaneous injection, degarelix was associated with significantly more injection-site reactions (pain, redness, and swelling) than leuprolide (40% vs <1%) and increased levels of liver enzymes in lab tests.

Anti-androgens

Anti-androgens block the body's ability to use any androgens. Even after orchiectomy or during treatment with LHRH analogs, the adrenal glands (glands situated above of both kidneys) still make small amounts of androgens. Drugs of this type, such as flutamide (Eulexin®), bicalutamide (Casodex®), and nilutamide (Nilandron®), are taken daily as pills. These drugs are generally added after treatment of bilateral orchiectomy in combination with LHRH analog in metastatic prostate cancer.

A standard treatment for advanced prostate cancer is androgen deprivation by surgical or medical castration. In theory, however, combined androgen blockade (CAB) with an antiandrogen plus castration should be more effective because castration alone does not completely eliminate androgens in the prostate. Therefore, a number of randomized clinical trials (RCT) were conducted in the 1990s to investigate the efficacy of CAB with an antiandrogen (nilutamide or flutamide) plus castration; however, there were both positive and negative results for the efficacy of CAB. The lack of data on safety, quality of life (QoL) and cost-effectiveness has been a hindrance to the adoption of CAB for the treatment of prostate cancer.

In the last few years, clinical research on CAB with the antiandrogen bicalutamide has started. CAB using this new antiandrogen was found to prolong overall survival in patients with prostate cancer, with favorable safety profiles and cost-effectiveness, without deteriorating QoL suggesting that CAB is a viable treatment option for prostate cancer when bicalutamide is used as the anti-androgen.

SIDE EFFECTS OF ADT

The use of hormonal therapy has a variety of adverse effects and they increase with the duration of the treatment. These side effects can include:

- Reduced or absent libido (sexual desire)

- Impotence (erectile dysfunction)

- Hot flushes, which may get better or even go away with time

- Breast tenderness, pain and/or gynecomastia (growth of breast tissue)

- Osteoporosis (bone thinning, porous and brittle) with greater incidence of bone fractures

- Anemia (low red blood cell counts)

- Decreased mental sharpness

- Loss of muscle mass

- Weight gain

- Fatigue

- Increased cholesterol

- Depression

Some research has suggested that the risk of high blood pressure, diabetes, strokes, heart attacks, and even death from heart disease is higher in men treated with hormone therapy, although not all studies have found this. Prolonged periods on hormone therapies for prostate cancer can result in osteoporosis. Annual dual-energy x-ray absorptiometry (DEXA) scans, also named bone density scans, are frequently used to screen for the development of osteopenia (lower bone mineral density) and/or osteoporosis measuring the patient's bone mineral density. DEXA is relatively easy to perform and the amount of radiation exposure is much less than a chest X-ray. The treatment with bisphosphonate has been demonstrated to reduce the risk of bone loss, but no guidelines currently exist for frequency of bisphosphonate administration.

Many side effects of hormone therapy can be prevented or treated. For example:

- Hot flushes can often be helped by treatment with certain antidepressants.

- Breast enlargement with radiation therapy.

- Osteopenia and/or osteoporosis with different biphosphonate medications

- Depression with antidepressants and/or counseling.

- Fatigue, weight gain, and the loss of bone and muscle mass with exercise or practicing a sport.

Secondary ADT

Estrogens (female hormones) were once the main alternative to bilateral orchiectomy for men with advanced prostate cancer. Because of their possible side effects (including blood clots and breast enlargement), estrogens have been largely replaced by LHRH agonists/antagonists and anti-androgens. Therefore, they are not recommend as initial therapy, but are frequently used after failure of the first line of treatment in metastatic prostate cancer patients together with anti-clotting drugs to prevent venous thrombosis (formation of a clot in the blood that either blocks, or partially blocks a blood vessel). Estrogens have similar side effects to ADT (see above). The main difference between them and bilateral orchiectomy is that anti-androgens may have fewer sexual side effects. When these drugs are used alone, libido and potency can often be maintained. When these drugs are given to men already being treated with LHRH agonists, diarrhea is the major side effect. Nausea, liver problems, and tiredness can also occur.

Ketoconazole (Nizoral®), first used for treating fungal infections, has been used in prostate cancer in combination with corticoid steroid since the mid-1990s. It is most often used to treat men recently diagnosed with advanced prostate cancer who have an extensive tumor burden, as it offers a quick way to lower testosterone levels. Ketoconazole can block the production of cortisol, an important steroid of the body. People treated with ketoconazole often need to take hydrocortisone, a corticosteroid, to prevent the side effects caused by low cortisol levels.

In April 2011, the FDA approved the androgen synthesis inhibitor, abiraterone acetate (Zytigac®), in combination with low dose prednisone (a corticoid steroid) for the treatment of men with metastatic castration-recurrent prostate cancer (CRPC) (see below) who have received prior chemotherapy containing docetaxel (Taxotere®). Abiraterone has been shown to shrink tumors, lower PSA levels, achieve better pain relief and help patients live longer. Doctors are now looking to see if this drug might be helpful earlier in the course of the disease as well. Treatment with abiraterone is well tolerated by patients. Side effects reported during its administration are swelling of the joints or discomfort, hypokalemia (low potassium in the blood), hypophosphatemia (low phosphate in the blood), edema (abnormal accumulation of fluid volume in tissues), muscle discomfort, hot flushes, diarrhea, dyspepsia, urinary tract infection, hypertension (high blood pressure), increase in liver enzymes and cardiac failure.

Xtandi® (MDV3100, enzalutamide) is a new antiandrogen that has recently been approved by the FDA (August 2012) for patients previously treated with docetaxel. In a phase III clinical trial, Xtandi increased the survival in CRPC patients by almost 5 months (18.4 months) compared with 13.6 months for those patients who received a placebo. The most common side effects of the drug are weakness, back pain, diarrhea, and pain in the joints.

TREATMENT OF CASTRATION-RESISTANT PROSTATE CANCER (CRPC)

Castration-resistant prostate cancer occurs in those patients whose disease continues to progress despite hormone therapy. CRPC requires documentation that the patient is medically castrate (serum testosterone below 50 ng/mL). By convention, CRPC is defined by a PSA rise of at least 2 ng/mL over the lowest castrate level of testosterone achieved during initial hormone therapy. Some patients will have cancer that relapses with rising PSA levels alone, others with increasing bone metastasis, and still others with a spread of cancer cells in other organs.

A number of options for systemic therapy should be considered based on the metastasis status. For CRPC patients without signs of distant metastasis but increasing the PSA levels, secondary hormone therapy is an option. Patients who are taking anti-androgen drugs like flutamide should discontinue the medication based on the observation that these agents contribute to the growth of cancer in later stages. A second hormone therapy, such as ketoconazole plus hydrocortisone or other estrogens, should be considered. None of these strategies has yet been shown to prolong survival and clinical responses, when they occur, are frequently short (between 2-4 months).

In 2010, the FDA approved sipuleucel-T (PROVENGE®) for the treatment of asymptomatic (showing no symptoms like pain) or minimally symptomatic metastatic CRPC patients. Sipuleucel-T is a dendritic cell vaccine generated from patients' peripheral blood mononuclear cells cultured with a human protein (PAP-GM-CSF) consisting of prostatic acid phosphatase linked to a granulocyte-macrophage colony-stimulating factor. The FDA approval was based on a phase III clinical trial. This study resulted in a 4.1-month improvement in median overall survival, 25.8 months compared with 21.7 months for placebo-treated patients, and an improvement in the rate of 3-year survival (31% versus 23%) in sipuleucel-T arm, with limited toxicity. Clinicians and patients should be aware that a decline in PSA and improvement in bone CT scans are not usually seen so fast as it has been hypothesized that immunotherapies take a longer time to work than other chemotherapy agents.

In cases of symptomatic disease showing signs of rapid progression or liver involvement or other soft tissue involvement, docetaxel (Taxotere®) with prednisone is the preferred first-line treatment. In 2004, the FDA approved such treatment on the basis of two large randomized trials (SWOG 9916 and TAX 327) comparing docetaxel-based therapy with mitoxantrone and prednisone in patients with CRPC. These trials demonstrated a significantly improved survival, with a median survival of 19.2 months for patients receiving docetaxel compared with mitoxantrone plus prednisone (16.3 months). Docetaxel was also superior to mitoxantrone with respect to pain response rate, PSA response rate, and improved quality of life. Based on these studies, the FDA approved the use of docetaxel together with prednisone as front-line therapy. Mitoxantrone combined with prednisone, which was approved before being superior to prednisone alone, became a second-line treatment for CRPC patients resistant to docetaxel.

Recently cabazitaxel (Jevtana®) was approved by the FDA for use in combination with prednisone for treatment of patients with metastatic CRPC previously treated with a docetaxel-containing regimen. The most common cabazitaxel adverse reactions include neutropenia (low white blood cells –neutrophils- count), anemia, Thrombocytopenia (low platelets count), diarrhea, fatigue, nausea, vomiting, constipation, asthenia (weakness), anorexia, peripheral neuropathy (functional disturbance of nerves), and alopecia (hair loss).

Currently, no consensus exists concerning the best second line therapy following docetaxel failure. Options include mitoxantrone, abirateone, docetaxel re-challenge, secondary ADT, sipuleucel-T and new drugs which have demonstrated a clinical benefit.

TREATMENT OF BONE METASTASIS

Bones are the most common site — in some patients the only site - of metastasis in most men with metastatic prostate cancer and these lesions can cause pain, debility, functional impairment, and lead to bone fractures with subsequent need for surgery and a preventive radiation therapy. Early detection of bone metastases can help determine the best treatment strategy. It can also help ward off complications. Because men with prostate cancer bone metastases often experience pain, pain management and improving their QoL are important aspects of all treatment strategies.

Treatment with bisphosphonates, denosumab and radioisotopes can help prevent complications related to bone metastases, like fractures. Bisphosphonates are drugs that are designed to help reset the balance in the bone between bone growth and bone destruction which is disrupted by the prostate cancer bone metastases. Zoledronic acid (Zometa®) is a bisphosphonate that can delay the onset of complications associated with prostate cancer bone metastases and relieve pain. Zometa was approved by the FDA in 2002. It is typically given once every three weeks as a 15-minute infusion. It is generally well tolerated. Potential side effects include kidney function problems and electrolytes (salts and minerals that can conduct electrical impulses in the body) imbalances.

Denosumab (Xgeva®) is a different type of bone-targeting drug which is given as an injection, rather than an infusion, and may be used instead of the zoledronic acid. There are some risks with both classes of bone-targeted agents, including something called osteonecrosis of the jaw (ONJ) that can occur after deep dental procedures or sometimes spontaneously. This can result in pain in the jaw and poor healing after dental procedure like extracting a tooth. Oral hygiene, baseline dental evaluation for high-risk patients, and avoidance of invasive dental surgery during the therapy are recommended to reduce the risk of ONJ. Daily calcium and vitamin D supplements are typically recommended to prevent hypocalcaemia (low calcium level in the blood) in patients receiving biphosphonates, and you should discuss this with your doctor. Zometa should be dose reduced in patients with impaired renal function and held for creatinine clearance < 30 ml/min.

Painful bone metastases can commonly be treated successfully with external beam radiation therapy. This generally involves 1-2 weeks of daily radiation treatments and can significantly improve symptoms. Sometimes radiation therapy may be recommended if there is an area of the bone (typically in the hip or leg) which looks as if it may easily break, even if it is not currently painful. The goal in that case is to reduce the risk of developing a fracture. This kind of radiation targeting sites of painful metastases can usually be safely given, even if you received radiation to treat your initial prostate cancer.

If there are multiple metastatic spots involved, medications called radioisotopes, also called radiopharmaceuticals, are often used. These radioactive isotopes can reduce pain in multiple spots all at once. A radiation oncologist injects the radioisotopes into a vein. The particles move through the blood stream until they concentrate in the areas of bone that contain cancer, where they deliver the radiation dose necessary to effectively irradiate the metastasis at a cellular level. The used radioisotopes include Samarium-153 and Strontium-89, both of which have been shown to effectively relieve pain caused by cancer metastases. The most commonly used agent is Strontium-89, which reduces pain in around 80 percent of patients. The side effects of radioisotopes are not frequent, but include fever, flushing, or a temporary pain in the bones. Their use is sometimes limited due to the fact that they can severely lower blood counts.

CONCLUSION

Men diagnosed with prostate cancer today have more therapeutic options than ever before. There is a number of new therapies that are in development. New chemotherapies, immunotherapies, targeted therapies like tirosine kinase inhibitors, vaccines, angiogenesis (formation of new blood vessels, especially blood vessels that supply oxygen and nutrients to cancerous tissue) inhibitors, and new radioisotope therapies are currently being tested in clinical trials. Some of these new agents will be approved soon to be used in prostate cancer patients.

RECOMMENDED PROSTATE CANCER WEB PAGES

Prostate Cancer Treatment Guide   www.prostate-cancer.com

Prostate Cancer Foundation   www.pcf.org

Prostate Cancer Foundation of Australia   www.prostate.org.au

Prostate Cancer Institute   www.prostate-cancer-institute.com

National Cancer Institute   www.cancer.gov/cancertopics/types/prostate

Prostate Cancer Canada   www.prostatecancer.ca

National Comprehensive Cancer Network   www.nccn.org